MURDER FOR STARTERS

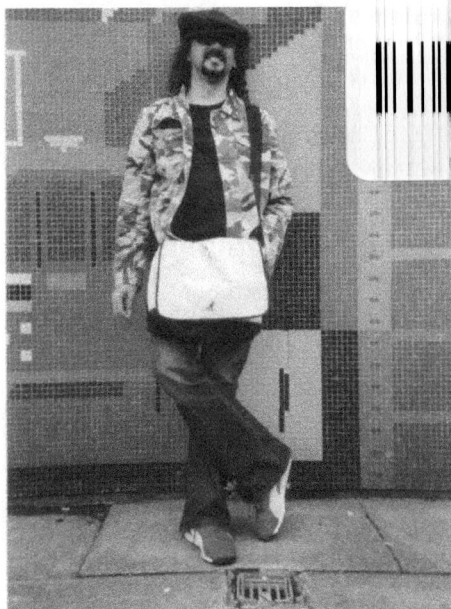

By Nick Satornetti-Portway

'One million people commit suicide every year.'
The World Health Organization

Published by
Chipmunkapublishing
PO Box 6872
Brentwood
Essex CM13 1ZT
United Kingdom

http://www.chipmunkapublishing.com

Proof-read by Michele Koh

Serial Killers-Therapists

Psssst wanna buy a second hand watch?
Sell me; tell me how do you feel…secretly
Reflective empathy-penetration, others other
Psychic clones of eugenic intolerance-branding
Al Capone-scarred mafia of spineless mothers-
pithed
Addled confused-hysterically-ideals of entry,
stiletto
Virginal monicled-wombed encouragement-
exposed
Introjected, splittists-eggs divided, self-squared
quarters
Projected contaminated-incompatibility, vaguely
spoken, whispers
Corruption-killers of corrugated fences-offended,
what sides Eden
Washing of karma hung dry or garrotted, sacrificial
bogman-tea stains

Infused engulfed Japanese mercurial
disfigurement-H, oblivions sure
Bloodied hands, cum in orgasmic denial of torture-
dun wid tea vicar
Kabbalistic Hitler fairies ring in Nebelung of lords
and ladies, timetable
Apartheid, Moses chosen sandals of bullock
manners-shi-Hittite soles
Lemon popsicles-communistic hatred-bedlam
borrowed-buskers wailing
Styx's remembered, pooh's toaistic-cormorants-
dying artless art
Monkey brains eschewed, swim bladder of warts
bursting kelp
Otter's brilliant sun, fashionable furs backed
sublime-crack
Mardi gra`s-bi-polars ice-en intuitive skidoo
Narwhales, walled whales
Vengeance of wrathful daggers, mind yourself-
gateless love

Masonic eyes cliqueyness, unarmed combat-
personality cult's impersonal personality
Touching perversity felt others-baize snookered
and scuppered, scuttling
Lagoons Friday-beauty, isolated in self
immolations, nobility's prized
Horizons blurred, vacuous embrace-plugged ears,
senseless death
Wounded, maggoted opened hearth-elastoplasts
un-naturalness, bound
Swerving streams consciousness, phobic
kindness of Lacananisms...
Nietzschian parties box, foolishly smiling-
imitations intimating truth
Mundane salami, bacchanalian deteoriation,
stoned jezebels-swelter
Judgemental statutes, torched money-green
goddess blackened
Engineered pavlovian behaviourist-latest, dead on
arrival, lost at sea

Chernobyl's egogic seclusion-purified in deathless
deaths, nettles grasped
Thingness-extracates tractions tractor of seeded
milarepa`s tome
Translators of kukurepa`s poisons bleached
peacocks-disembowelled
Ophelia's seared heart-dried blood exhumed
teeth-"rang jung"
Dawns faded clouds strike swansong in measured
joy, joyfully
Consummated Satsuma, ippon`s kimono, shellac
embellished heart
Staggered facet, masked guilt of executioner's
songstress-butterfly fish
Pinned voodoo, therapists myxamatosis-burnt
offerings honoured
Big Mac's superficial clown, crowned in hell
realms chasm of pleasurable pain.
Frenzies of zombies' breath, extinguished life's
love-nailed Hawaiian hooped corpses
Sequentially sequential.

Beginning-less Birth of No Birth

When did I begin, to dance in infinity?
A thought from being of thought of being
Conceptual madness, idea of no idea of ideas
Chicken without an egg, egg without a chicken
Cosmic whirlpool stirred, naked atoms of dustless
dust
Stoked voided fires, darkened sun of no son,
eclipsed
Uterine rivers coursed, Milky Way of no-way of the
way
Umbilical strangle hold of deathlessness of life-
nourished
Breathlessly drowning for rebirth of no birth of birth
Centreless centre of no edge of edge of
edgelessness
Penetrated black hole, sucked inside out, of
outside in

Vision's bursting eyes plucked; holiness's filth-
divinely divine
Luminosity burns the darkened pyre-suttee
devoured flesh
Sacrifice of no sacrifice, subjected submission
elevated
Sell every cell of cellular space of no space-
expanded
Divide and conquer, split asunder, spiritual waters
of chromosomes
Daybreak and breath-pain seers my eyes, colours
washed rainbows
Touching tenderly painfully unreal reality of
delusional illusion
Journey of no journey's pathless path travelled,
but where is no where
Thoughtless energy absorbed and dissolved
transcended clouds cloud
Swimming in inhospitable hospitality-leached lies
drunk-universal love

Expanded expansion of no expansion is to love
the love of love, love
Where do we end, but begin in beginingless end
of no end to begin
Finger were do you start but end and write of
writerless thoughts
Inklessly darkened lightened consciousness,
oneness of one of no-one, but one
Birth, but where should I begin in
begininglessness of no being begin.

Airless Grass of Cutty Sark

Paper sky cranes in its decline of blue
Mirrored crystal foolishly jests at wisdom
Thunderbolts dragon scorches stupidity
Pools of bracken haven, gorse gallops
Amazingly burnt amber stares at death
Detritus flowers in defiance of the sun
Thread of braided silken meadows-weave
Water falls and fails in love of stonewalls
Fodder of parchment unwritten formulation
Bacteria of mathematical holiness squared
Phoenix enviously pursues Agni`s children
Styx of galleon executes simplistic Vetch
Framed birth eggs the tormentor of seconds
Dissolving oneness in abjection of life-endless
Algae's dustless lust, leached consciousness
Shrunken Luna expanse-devoid of breath
Shrouded imprinted perception contaminated
Golden greens the view of deforested attachment
Yamataka stirs blackness of lighted visions spiral

Diamond garland bequeathed, decapitated fragrance
Intoxicated nothingness extinguishes no-thing, voided.

Apologies For Living

I would like to apologise,

For my life as and of a lie
Gene's no-one would wear
My father gentle, uneducated
My mother intoxicatingly stupid,
In her intellectual aggression
Misunderstood in being
But being another's genes, of
Non acceptance in any form
But what is form?
Except acceptance
Recognised in unrecognition
To exist in absence
Of non existence of absence
Bereft of substance
Except genes of mass productions
Couplings of neverness
Painful realities genes

Provoke me to provoke

Could I sue for life's genes?

Take them back, refunded

Discarded torn lifelessness

Patched others blue genes

I am not considered worthy

Wanderer's vagabond's thing

Speechless in contaminations genes

But what size is right

None at all fit

Unisex

Masculine, femininity

Intellectual

Thicko

Lover of so much

Falseness or truth

Thief

Compassionate

Kindliness

Killer

Rescuer

Honest to lie

Blinded

Visionary

Sexual provocateur

Tender otherliness

Mirror of my own ugliness

But a mirror of others beauty

Intuitive awareness

Dumbed silence

Reprisals

Revenge

To love is unforgivable

But to love, oh love

My genes need washing

Intolerable unacceptence

Stains of penetration, otherliness

Is this love?

Genes of jealousy

Genes of hatred

Sickness of sicknesses

Condemned for my blue genes

What genes would you wear?

I wear the genes of death

The mockers of genetics

Hazel eyes that should be scorched

Because they see, but to see

These genes of isolations islands?

Abandoned blue genes, in windy washing lines

Unfortunate genes

Would you buy my genes?

For sale, genes;

Of a loveless life

So I apologise

For my genes

My life,

Apologies,

Apologies, apologies-sorry.

Bag of Diseased Love

Bag of diseased love-disillusioned youth
Eyes poisoned beauty-suffocation
Trembling innocence-sacrificed heart
Heedless intoxication-numbed emotions
Equatorial amniotic fluid-fills earthen ears
Habituated thinking-experienced cyclic motion
Ego's construction company-defended bloodied
river
Ocean of bodies lap at the shore of oblivion

Birdless Thoughts

Bird of thought, glides in sky of blue

Clouds of nuances, darken the sun

Rain of reason, emotional cyclone-swirls

Lightning's wisdom, scorched earth-touched

Fruited tree of fruitless love-infestation of desire

Falling thought, discarded leaves-golden scythe

Seeds of infinity, abstraction of fertility

Planted femininity, receptive waters

Numerous atoms, attract to distract

Poisonous gas, anaesthetized heart

Rock of no rock, disintegrating flesh

Suicidal swifts digest macabre fleetings

Wingless idea, drowns-depth of no depth

Solar storm, irradiated eyes-visionless vision

Ebb and flow of beauties shore-washed moon

Quadruped's twofold conscience-awakened dawn

Flowering knowledge of boundless edge-timeless

Imploded universal thought of no thought-extinct

Death of no death, beginingless streams-
meanderings, where
Birdless thought, existence of no existence-
thinking died, to-day!

Black Solitary Chrysanthemum

Loneliness, my faithful companion, always
Intimate lover, never rejecter nor neglecter
Foreshadowed shadow casts her black love
Into encapsulated hollow tender heart, beautiful
Loving pain of love, soaked bloodless body
Starved of love, yet loved lovelessly
Loneliness touches my breast, kisses my inner
kiss
Wrap yourself in & around me, delusional love of
love
Knowledge of her darkness profoundly illuminating
Prostituting loneliness, lover unbound unwanted
Desiring yearning her second by second, infinitely
Yet only for separation, cruelty tearing my love
from love
I can not betray her, yet who would believe, I
could
Joined at birth, my incestuous sister loneliness
Suckled and tasted the same milky breath

Caress the same sheets; hug the same pillow, as each;

Dies and dies in the others loneliness of loneliness

Surrendering surrender to her once again

Come to my bosom and our bed, share pleasurable pain

It will not be long before, death arrives,

We will be together, forever,

Loneliness and I.

Blackened Love

Black angel

Sings

Biting frost

Gangrenous heart

Aggression filters through

Savage stance

Flames boil up

Breathless spite

Love dies

A thousand deaths

In frustration

I count grains of sand

The desert bloom

Has cracked

Camel spit

The only nourishment

Barren love

Laughs no-more.

Blackest of Night

Black black secret
Black night
Bring your wing
Across the daylight
As the day is
Set to rest
We are blessed
With the opalescence
Of the moon
To fill our womb
With granite like grey
For we obey
The law of day
The dark
Has made its mark
Instilling in our heart
A sense of fear
Because loved ones are not near

Alone we fight

Our darkest foe

Which is our own mind

As we are not kind

And slow

To take heed

Of our greatest deed

That troubles us so

When we are low

Black black night.

Brown Sugar Sky

Veils of mist

Hang heavy

As I chase it

Down a silver valley

Inhaling the clouds

As the fire burns

Run dragon run

Hazy view

As my body becomes numb

My mind is sent

To euphoric heights

Honeydew sun

Seductive copper brown

Skin rough to the touch

Head of vivid green

Waves goodbye

In the midday breeze

Black winged angels

Appear in flight

Against a palette of blue and white

Calling in a strange cacophony

Disappearing

Into a gossamer filled sky

As quickly as they come

Grasshoppers sing

As lightening lizards

Bask on a rock

Waiting for their chance

As my mind fades

Sleep creeps over me

As a snake slips

Into the grass

Day has gone

Forever long

Buddha's Moondust

The heaviness of the moondust clinging to the snowdrops humbling stance is the presence of you my love our love, the fields of snowdrops bow as compassion out weighs the pains of histories karmic accumulations of precious rebirths each pollinated by the bee of compassion in its unfurling of wisdom's stream, the streams of nectar, the centre of the lotus blossoms blossoming enlightened activity the light of love..................which hurts my eyes.............the hazel of the coppices brow...........the brow of the furrowed earth...........the worm of enquiry..................pertains to the gurus smile the sun and moon of completeness the eclipse of hearts and minds entwined in the dance of the double helix the serpentine caudices of the feminine goddess's lightening bolts the meteoric sacredness of the Garuda's path in its flightless path to the sanctity of the speech of the airless quality of divine presence the Buddha, the enlightened activity of the luminous nature of universal reality each as it is as suchness of blissfulness`s presence the atoms of containment and the interconnected nature of all creation ever present, knowable in an instant...........................the all encompassing enlightened activity of a Buddha, emaho.

"Buy My Book?" (Bejan Matur)

I will not buy your book?
I will kiss your heart!
Walls are dust-speaking to me
Speechlessly,
Spreading flowers-touching sea's
Seeds fruitlessly baring the sun
Clouded reasons are no-reason to hail
Worldliness's heartlessness is its heart
Islands of landlessness`s land in no-land
Netted sights wanderings, in-between
Mountains of genetics, smelting forests
Purities extracted instinct-decomposed
No-mad`s man is motherlessly listlessly lost
Earthen pot, shattered gourd, waterless tears
Encampments burnt in exiled minds eyes
Gaseous death smoulders in nostrils of tundra
Bricks kill in blind buildings of emptiness
Confetti of bodies, sweeping streets

Of;

Darkened breeze of loving hands
Earthliness is barren of soiled love
Patient weavers, threadless fingers
Aprons cooking in boiled vinegar of
Mustards entrenched air of airless airs air.
Every day's day is my people's pain, today's day.

To the Kurdish people and all oppressed people,
everywhere.

Coated History

History wears you like a leather glove

Tough but with soft malleable fingers

Worn down to transparency

As war bleeds tips of intolerance

With trigger happy hatred

Waves pound your conscience

Never to be halted

Kanute drowns in predigest and pride

As sand bleaches the hairs of time

In sectarian punishment; lies

Fathoms deep

In blue black discrimination

Silt stirs the dregs of humanity

Clogged gills suffocate in the breath of life

Hearts, beliefs, buried beneath

Powdered ashen love; blown in the wind

To touch is to destroy; fragility unbounded

Corn Plasters and Kisses

I sit here contemplating you in a smile of moonflakes trembling in droplets of dew hanging from gossamer threads over a golden hued earthen clay pot standing by the steps of the gate into my orchard as dusk settles in dusts lament of fading rays of light scattered by nights arrival at the non arrival of you as croaking chorus's of heartened joyful other cascade in me, oh you my love what and were.......thinking the thought that could be you or even us, to dress you in your naked awareness that dances in vibrations of rippling scent of senselessness in the view of nonview that seers my sight in sightless you in essence the taste of the wind rustling in footsteps upon brittle egoless leaves crumbling hearts of infused tealess stains that lie in my cup, I hold touchingly closer to my breast in a sighed release in the illuminated you, the moth battling in its ardour at its misguided flame snuffed in an instant of rainbow dreams of non existence in existence but to exist is not but you.........the warmth of your flesh against mine burns the cool night air in its openness in expanded expansionless`s expansion in chasm's chamber the prisoner of your hand held in mine, your eyes floweringly brutal in glances of tenderness in and of imagined love kissing my lustless sex of passionless passion of our wombed worldless world in its worldliness of unworldliness to love, the love for you my Shadowless one, kissing your pathless path to blissfulness`s bliss of sweet rain quenching my thirst in you and of you, my love......... the clouds of doubt enliven me in you my love, my love.

Dakini`s Tears

Dakini`s tears, the turquoise lake
Heart drops of dzi, the necklace of obtainments
Tso Pema, fire of the Lotus born, the unborn
dance
Tears and nectar the spindle of compassion
The primordial essences of mirror like wisdom
The Pearls of sound, universal display defiled
emptiness
Om, Mandarava grant your blessings
The rain of compassion, the jewels of wisdom
The dew on the petal of existence, Om Chenrezig
Oh compassionate one, the one whose smile,
destroys illusions
The tears of Vajrayogini`s skullcup, the blessings
of immortality
The melodious sweet jewels of the Ani la`s
butterlamp
The fire of my hearts compassion, oh Dakini bless
me

I supplicate the body of existence and the death of
egogic pain
You, oh enlightened Mandarava, destroyer of
Mara's hoards
The demonic heretics, the corrupters of minds
stream essences
Kukurepa`s libation, the poisonous tears, the bitch
of mortality,
The bag of pus and water, our attachments to bile
and piss
The body of the cotton clad one, oh heretical saint,
teach
The Dakini`s tears of wisdom and compassion
I supplicate to the holy Dharma the law beyond all
laws
The light the of unborn nature of
Samatrabhadra and Samatrabhadri the union of
non-union
The tears of universal compassionate sound,
The love of the universal Dakini, pearls of wisdom

The scatterings of Lotus petals, oh bless this
ground
Mother earth the Dakini of our birthless birth
The flower of existence, Tara's manifestation of
lotus light
Grant the Om of our tears the supplication of life's
light
The sacred sacredness of sound, the heart drops
of Dharmakhaya
Grant your blessings oh holy sadhu,
Fishgut eater cast your net of non-compassionate
compassion
The Zangpo of primordial waters, supplications of
the wombless womb
The Dakini`s tears, the feminine divine, the hand
of kindness
I supplicate, divine mother of all Pranaparamita
Buddha nature, the Dorje Chang of spaciousness
The sky of supplications, the tears of the Dakini,
Om ah hung,
Hri.

Damaged Strange Love.

Saw you in the mall,
Amongst the apples
Green soft bodied
Hidden and hidden
Yet not hidden
Wings transparently delicious
Stocking thinned legs
Six in all, my lucky number
You looked half dead
Suffocating sterility
Chemicals to stop
Rotten blackened taste
The taste of your
Dying odour
Drenches my
Sense, love

Oh strange fly
Come lie,

With me, in hand

Love, resuscitate

Your damage

And be

Free.

Love for a stranger.

budwaria3.

Dancing in the Flames-Lovelessly

Wisdom dances-burning fleshless desires
Moon embraces her cold fireless heart
Stars subdue the grief in her eyes,
Universe within universe-cries voided
Meteorically metal encloses her being
Body of no body-macabre purity sullified
Flowing endlessly to beginingless end
Fiercelessly entwined essence within essence
Love of no-love is the endless love-her
Petrifies my bones kissing my mind numblessly
Bleached black-spinelessly grasping emptiness
Life of flowering supernova-exploding
expansiveness
Saturations spiralling beauty-evasively she
dissolves
Wisdoms tender smile-gently devours my head
Rational of no head heedlessly dies of love in love
of love
Ballerina of worlds, swan bows before white light

Searing love opens my chest, cavity of hate-extinguished

Cranes sore across skyless bluebirth of no birth-to birth

Within her she permeates my softness to painful reality

To die the death of no death her touch seductively wise

To remember is to forget her-ever present presence

Wrathful lips pierce my anger-subdued degradation

Washes darkened heart-lovelessly kindness shines

Rebirth in totality of reality is to love-endlessly

Burningly she kills with compassionate wisdom;

Dakini drink of me-bloodlessly divine wisdoms fire-embraced

To dance the dance of no dance endlessly expanding nakedness

Awareness of her is to die in the furnace of loving flames-wisdom.

Darkness Enfolded

Confusion, illusion, delusion; reality understated

Shards of coloured light, hit my retina

As day becomes night, black pit

Elevated above mother, knarled wood

Blind love stumbles around, sees nothing

Serpent woman rises, conception perceived

Rock spirit smashes my face, into a billion pieces

Rush of air, bequeaths me

Decapitated darkness, knives cut out stillness

Stimulation, devoid of nature

One taste, all powerful

Crystallised vision, burns bright

Sexuality entices, desires bow to seduction

Mournful queen, macabre stain

Release me, into the zenith

Of all encompassing sun

Freedom sharply sliced

Solitude no more

Life eternally, revealed.

Death's Exquisite Kiss

Death's silhouette steely embraces me
Collapsing on a bed of puritanical snow
Holly bushes drip blood fruit
Rattling voice, I beckon him closer
Ashen cold lips tenderly touch mine
Frosty passion, my mortal blow
Clicking bony hands, grasp my breast
Excited, my heart stops
His coldness, enters me
Decreasing cloudy vision,
Death's beautiful face;
Darkness revisited
Annihilated warmth
I reach
Orgasmic consciousness's release
Massacred breath leaves me
In deaths final,
Exquisite kiss.

Delusional Reality

GOD,

Who is GOD?

I am God

Am I one with GOD?

Or am I actually GOD?

Germ of reason, irrational reality

Is GOD dead-mortal remains, cosmic implosion?

Nietzsche knew

Did he die in me?

Or did I kill him?

Lack of love, for him or me; possibly

Is this reality, or am I deluded

When was his funeral?

Last century; I wasn't invited

Was it a secret; it must have been

Some still believe, because it was a secret, maybe

Who created who?

GOD created man,

Or did man create God?

Is this sanity or insecure delusion?

Am I going mad?

Stalin, Hitler, Mao, Pol Pott;

Devils with the power of a GOD

Millions cut down with the sickle of hate

Mowing the lawn, English past time

Or was it fate- Determinism?

GOD culling the race; Dolphins, Elephants

Sacrifice; GOD to GOD

Sacrificed GOD of irrationalities, tarred and feathered

More acceptable

Is this reality or delusional?

Is life of any value; personally, universally?

GOD knows

Or does he?

If we don't; all hell will be let loose!

Possibly or has the worst already happened?

Devilish….. Bondage

Complement me daaarling!

Do you like?

My breasts!

Are they?

Young;

Soft, firm and sweet,

Devourer them,
Heartily,
Take handfuls,

Deliriously drink;
From the…
Trough of,

Fleshful desire.

Sinner!

Satiate yourself,

Further;

With nipples,

Yearning to be;

Sucked, tongued,
Mouth-saliva, trickling,
Twisted sugar candy,
Teethed and nibbled,

Until;

I'm wet,

Butter melting....

Darling is;

Aaron's rod,
Golden and long?

Pointing to;

The Gods-above.

Let my lily white;
Hands........... extend,
Curling slender;
Fingers,

Grasp!

Electricity;
Lights up the,

Darkness.

Subjugate……………yourself,

Kneel before;

My open…….
Wound;

Purse………..

Your………..Lips;

Tenderly,

Kiss,

The reddened;

Raven,

And;

Die………

As I,

Bury………

You're…….

Head;

In…………

My Earthen………

GRAVE.

Dumbed Speechlessness of Heartfelt Joyful Bliss.

Heartless hearts joyfulness is the smile that caresses others
Speechlessness of speech in the speech of no-speech but love
To touchingly touch divine tenderness is to open like a flower
Drinking from the sun supping the nourishment of breastless wisdom
Nectar's suffocation is as a bee intoxicates the hivelessness of the hive
Dancing in directionless directions pathless path to blissfulness
To dance is to pluck the soft clouds reign of contentment in poverty
Otherliness floatlessly breathes the breathless vision of blindness
Amber's concealed earthiness is entombed in doubtless doubt of doubt

Living is to flow in estuaries meeting of seas,
mingling droplessly in droplessness
Soundlessly eons counting eons of eons in
infinities embraceless embrace
Spacious blackness of the avoided voided
emptiness of emptiness is emptiness
Deathlessness of masked death is appealingly
dying to see realities unreality
Scented scentlessness the arrow maker's fragrant
fragrance occupies my heart
Monsoons bathing in gutterlessness of guttural
toned deafness vibratingly joyful
Garbage heaped in nothingness but obsessive
wealthless wealth of worthlessness
Meteorically compounded chasms receptiveness
courses the heavens rustiness
Blacksmith bellows a wrathful heatless heat of
forged totality in everything
Atomless atoms of spiralling cosmos enshrines
the gateless gate of no-gate

Entering the entertainment of non-entertainment is
entering the entrance of no-entrance
To enter the womblessness of wombed
wombness is to be the sky, oh cloudy
cloudlessness`s cloud.
Blotted speech is the speech of speechlessness of
listening silence in silence.

Earth Bound Love

Brittle heart drowns,
In an ocean of neglect
Mother, love me, love me

Talons of scarred disease
Painful forest of isolation
Mother, love me, love me

Abandoned youth
Dejected hope
Mother, love me, love me

Blackened eyes seethe
In beautiful disgrace
Mother, love me, love me

Jealous icy breath
Consumed breast
Mother, love me, love me

Hateful tormented being
Devoured flesh of flesh
Mother, love me, love me

Violence concealed in
Ashen cloak of death
Mother, love me, love me

Love me, love me.

Eternal Punishment-Madness.

Damnations, raining heavy atoms,

Cyclical tormentors ascended

Limb fighting limb,

Pruned clipped fingers;

Leprosy mindlessly grasps

Discarded shredded self-worthlessness

Possessed falseness attacks;

Demonic faceless memory

Confronted presence projected

Tearing fleshless hatred, seething

Scorched silhouette, blackened vision

Inner landscape-devastated wasteland

Disembodied, becomes bodied other

Destructive despising queen burns white hot;

Raw open wounds, diseased loveless sanity

Haunted, reasonable rejecter, negativity

Degradated painful tender heart, cries;

Molten veined Mother earth, torturer

Miasmic foggy oblivion, released torrent

Stalking blindfolded rationality, mirrored
Instinctual insight, penetrates superficiality
Drowning in shallowness of life, madness
Detested historical abusiveness, peeled open
Virulent aggression, mentalities assassin's
Scarred psychic matter, bloodless revelation
Surgically removed repugnant egotistical tissue
Timeless healer, shroud and infuse my soul;
Miracles and magic are prophesised,
Transcended pinnacle, liberated being
Embrace's the love of love, to love;
Unconditionally;
Is madness mad of madness?

Yes my love, to love we go!!

Even if………………..

Even if there is no sun, there is still warmth

Even if there are no clouds, there is still softness

Even if there is no sea, there is still a shore to
meet

Even if there is no earth, there is still ground to
stand on

Even if there is no rain, there is still sustenance

Even if there is no light, there is still clarity

Even if there is no wind, there is still air to breathe

Even if there is no food, there is still nourishment

Even if there is no flesh, there is still being

Even if there is no vision, there is still sight

Even if there are no friends, there are still
companions

Even if there are no parents, there are still routes

Even if there is no love, there is still compassion

Even if there is no rhythm, there is still dancing

Even if there is no movement, there is still life

Even if there is no knowledge, there is still wisdom

Even if there is no fruit, there is still abundance

Even if there is no marriage, there is still togetherness

Even if there is bondage, there is still freedom

Even if there is no money, there is still wealth

Even if there is no structure, there is still form

Even if there is no ego, there is still presence

Even if there is no position, there is still a point

Even if there is no view, there is still a horizon

Even if there is no beauty, there is still joy

Even if there is no happiness, there is still laughter

Even if there are no boundaries, there is still containment

Even if there are no thoughts, there is still self

Even if there is no soul, there is still spirit

Even if there are enemies, there is still no hatred

Even in extreme pain, there is still love, love and love, to love.

Evenings Drunken Lightless Light

A palanquin winds around undrenched Ganga's flowers floating thoughts bloated in unrealities reality, camen nibble at shrouded eyes, teeth boned in muddied Sadhu bathed in filth of purities pollutants of contaminated temples sandless libations of nectar's wisdom, Dakini bleeds in renewal of days cowed in eclectic rhythmic moonless joy, dewless blossoms clouds sky in deathless Taj Mahal of marbled scent bleaching the earth, lightening spiders in parasol of blisslessness's bliss to kiss the steps of Bodhgaya in homage of emptiness of formless form in emptiness's careless caress raining immortal nectar of hooded ribbed cage of abandoned defencelessness's defences to open hearted universal grief in the love of grieving love, to love but die in spaciousness's space is expanded expansion of expansionlessness expansioness of infinities infinity of begininglessness beginning of endlessness of no point in pointless view of non view but of viewless view, buying nothing but dusty eons of birthless birthed flowered blissfulness pollinated in a suns breast of rubbled flesh grinding bones of karmic retribution dissolving in dissolution of dissolving ignorance of ignorant unreality of realities mundane truth of luminosities relativeness of unrelative relativity of relative truth of no truth but truth of truth.

Evenings Spacious Morning, You My Love

Birdlessness of thoughtless thoughts is of you and
in you, love
Touching spacious blues fleshless clouds the
breath of your eyes, is you
Wind of warming suns, freshness of breast, is
cusped mouthingly in you
Willow of hands seductively melt ravines of
curvaceousness, is of you, in you, love
Enfolding, grasplessly embracing snowy
mountains of you and in you, is you, love
Compassionate orgasms ascendance of raindrops
affections is of you and in you, love
Kissing nakedness of berries reddened lips,
tango's `n salsa's in you and of you, love
Trainless rivers reaching in oceanics
oceanlessness of you, oceans of you, is you, love
Evaporation in sparinglessness`s absorption of
softened love, is you and of you, love

Peached moon eclipsing wisdoms passionless
passion of you, is you and of you, love
Savannahs lushness of fleeting flowers is you and
of you, my love, you, us
Wildly calm childless light in wilderness of
otherliness, is you, of you, love
Pollinating mindlilessness of mind in you and of
you, is us, love-oneness my love
Walled skin of no skins, boundaries of no
boundaries traversed, is you and of you, love
Heartless joy of hearts entwining, blisslessly divine
bliss, is you and of you, my love
Meeting in forgetfulness's remembrance to be with
you and of you, is you, my love, us
Namelessness of named, but not named is you
love, my love, you of you, us love
Carriageless carriages window of concealed
compartment is exposure of you, you my love, us
Loveless love of you is the you of no you but us,
nothingness`s emptiness, love my love, love.

Fleeting Warmth, Sea of Contact

Wind blown leaves, rustling
Down the streets of London
Life's path- staggeringly painful.

Love reaches out to;
Stranger, encountered,

Openness expands;

A smile exchanged
Warmth of eyes, shine
Lovingly, words of interest
Melt away differences
Soft peach of conversation, dances
Laughter, flowering blissful sun
Momentary aeons of space
Seconds, minutes, evaporate
Time doesn't exist,
Present, joyfully explored!

Until;

We
Depart, separate,
Dissolve into crowded life

Heart full of other,

Fleeting warmth,
Sea of contact,

Washes away, attachment

Wind blown leaves, rustling
Down the streets of London
To-day is every day, beautiful joy.

God/Devil Are One………..

Light and dark

Good and evil

Man and woman

Beauty and ugliness

Parent and child

Happiness and sadness

Teacher and pupil

Guru and student

Master and slave

God and the Devil

Heaven and earth

Above and below

Sinner and saint

Dirty and clean

Right and wrong

Negative and positive

Microcosm and macrocosm

Chaos and order

Spirituality and sexuality

Rational and irrational

Sanity and madness

Wisdom and stupidity

Nirvana and samsara

Weakness and strength

Cause and effect

Beginning and end

All have been separated

Far, far too long

Whatever your beliefs

We are one

Heal the divide

Each is one and the same

No opposites,

No subject, object

No Karma

Symbiotic oneness,

We are one,

Oneness in love

Humanity, universe

One Love.

Headlessly Heading in Headlessness`s Head

Corn's dry rustling is quenched by sunless
warmth's sun
Grass's verglessly scattering the path of
joyfulness`s joy
Flamelessly your breathless hairless air's golden
light;
Drenches the breeze of your presence's
presencelessness
Habituated hearts habitless habit is inhabited in
habit's heart
Bloodless water bleeds in streams of crystalline
rainbows
Colourless colour paints the palate of your eye's
gaze
Softening clouds of delight in tender embraces of
forgetfulness's:
Naked arboratorium in palanquins of awareness's
enclosed expansiveness

Spaciously skyless skies spaciousness is
emptilessly empty of you
Presence's presence's of presence is
presencelessness of your touching
Swaves of swirling stars dance in endless dances
of dancing loveless love
Wheels of time spin in timelessness`s time, but to
begin......were
Soaked tealess tea of ceremonies in eons of love,
lightless light-bathes you're.....
Singing flowers crumple in expressions expression
of life's lifeless life
Sweep the night-sky in dustlessness`s dust of
bargained rational-bartered
To breathe is to breathe in breathless`s breath of
otherliness`s other other
To you my love shine as you've never shined
before-shinelessly shine and shine!

Happy birthday love.
Thanx,Nick Satornetti-Portway.

Hypocrisy-Denuded Death

Red sky hangs heavy, blood soaked clouds-dripping

Fractural of barren wasteland, de-fleshed trees-stairway climbed

Poisonous breathe of lungless love, suffocated intoxication-induced

Desire of no-desire is no-desire of desire, extinction of sound-deafens

Tear washed earth, diluted sea of silted thermal vents-boiled

Stifled white heat-submerged sustenance, suckling pig roasted

Chilled day, salutes the enemy-she has arisen, in denial of denial

New born flowers, devoured petal by petal, scented fruit-deseeded

Decomposed thought, constructed composition composted, steaming dew

Ethereal vision of no vision, darkened seminal light-glistening bacteria

Being of no-being is being, molecular chromosome, Zested bath digested

Plucked heart sustained, gods draw water in the air-emaciated love

The He of no-one touches the scarecrow of Indian solace-marooned monsoon

Saffron of vegetated dis-ease, sublimated Smokey eyes-cushioned throne

Fleeced of golden thread, salted corn, eclipsed-beautiful similes of opalescence

Graded grains counted, rivulets trickle down breasted snow geese, frightened flight

Umbilical of girthed fertility pierced, ricochet of fire, burnt sterility crumbles

Tabled mountain furnished in gaping chasm of yore, fountain of ambrosial youth-quenched

Dreamed rainbows breached, disembowelled sarcophagus, enshrined language

Deciphered being deconstructed, icicle berries burst asunder, hieroglyphic scars

Romanised dolphin surfs imaginary waters-clay octopus's fluidity, grasped blackly

Sparse maple pans fluted coliseum of polluted nightshades mirrored eyes

Brittle urchin walks the bodiless Judas tree of snakeweeds laced wings

Harpy eagle rips chattering minds chains of deceitful tenderness, scuttled

Descended flycatcher sawlessly faces the portraiture of pain-swamped

Mosquitoes probe chambers of quatrain's mafia cellophane caged thylacine

Scrofula enacted retreat of hysterical hyena, paces the circumference of circumstance

Infinite zero transcends logic of Pre-Raphaelites hated love-lustless poppy bled

Trigonometry conveys flying fishes released regalia of echolalia`s ecad

Until eclectical demise of nihilism's demonised hippocampus-dies in sludge.

My Briefness of Lizzy.

Your disfigured damaged fleshless wound could not conceal the love of and for you, those eyes that beaconed me from the hell of your car park recognised and yet not recognised, your path danced towards life in a deathlessness of waiting and wanting in an alcove of exposure of travelling tenderness awkwardly sharing your joyless insights of mannerisms of a wombless child, to eat from your plate was not hard, but so painfully real to see your wings tethered to the earth wanting to fly off and in my thoughtless thoughts of personal desire yet of no-desire, is my damnation of your damnation in recognised damnation of lightless love, to release a heavy heart that hung in the balance of timelessness of endless time but no time, arriving and arrived to soon, to soon, to soon.

Love Carnivorous Embrace.

Melting my eyes into your flesh
Delectable bloodless flowers
Blooming soft buttercup cheeks
Crimson breasts sipped deliriously
Limbs of green mould breathed
Lichen of shoulders arched gateway
Arboretum of heart felt desire mused
Peaches of buttocks, bruising fingers
Handless crescent caress browed sky
Feetless feathered calf swans down
Boundaries curvaceous chestnut
Clam like

Love Cleansed

Tenderly she rises, opening her petal's to embrace the light, hair knotted eyes-dewy cotton, closely clinging sweated breasts, moons joyful lustfully lost shadows, perused thoughts-darkened horseless rhythm, deserted heart-swallowed shores, pounding limbless surf-foamed desire, mirrored yesteryear washed facial memories, seaweeds amazed fond, bursting with contact, touched cheek, snow melted lips dripped bloodless berries, mouthed reality experienced, taste of no taste-tasted, but is it love? Pollen showered body, clouded view, steamed lashes caress follicles barren waning skin, shrouded bladed torso coiled fingers, towelled gentleness, blessed feet, cloven luck-despondent look at life, marrowed marriage, boned friendless cave, raging fire, embers ignite passionless passion, fruit peeled and sliced, seeds-world in palm of hand, sparkling marooned lagoon, Jupiter spun web, entombed delirious scentless bed-entrapped rapture fractured, boundlessly blissful crumbling ego, humility bows to earthen teacher-clay pigeon shot sky, cunningly steals her night, gales thrash her mind, weather-drummed hail, beaten anvil, silver and gold threaded spirit-levels the pain she feels, mortar pocked enemy, exploding addiction-attachment nullified, Spartan language fed, wisdom's kiss is unutterable joy-tenderly she rises, in my bosom!

Love The Conqueror.

Love is the conqueror and the concubine

Its breath delights the budding flowers

Its honey subdues the sting of desire

Spaciously love fills all emptiness

The starless star is the brilliance of;

The smile of the Dakini`s touchless touch

The breastless sun is warmly felt, ashen

The dew is the water of loving love

The petal of supplication, elevates my love

The liberator of libations, love in its loveless love

The sound of her, love............... lovingly love

Relentless as the oceans of abandonment

The sea of fulfilment, loves lovingly, love

The cup, the hand, the non-clasping love, of love

The lighted love that blinds in its radiance, the

release.......love

Yet to love is, the all................. Lovingly love,

love

To love lovelessly loving love, love.

Love Carnivorous Embrace.

Melting my eyes in your flesh
Delectable bloodless flowers
Blooming soft buttercup cheeks
Honeyed breasts sipped deliriously
Limbs of green mould breathed
Lichen of shoulders arched gateway
Arboretum of heart felt desire mused
Peaches of buttocks bruising fingers

Loves Down Cast Shadow

Shackled societies negative thoughts-
Pessimistic soaked freedom
We edged between door of,
Spiralling conflict
Blinded eyes see the sound of
Choked innocence's last breath;
Squeezed out.
Pain dies in a trickle of salty tears
Weapons disfigured face, laughs
As love falls under the black sun
Hateful joy burns,
Wealth of children's bodies
Tortured vivacity abounds
In minds bloodied hand
Scattered flesh martyred
In a wasteland of intolerance
Love is consumed in,
Death's shadow
Annihilated heart.

Loves Exerted Death

Crumpled dead butterfly wing
Breathless breeze caresses my heart
Haunted dust lies in life's empty shadow
Voices soundlessly echo
In space of chastisement
Death's obsolete statue reinvents itself
Bloated bruised lips, sip its sweetness
Michelangelo's beauty, transfigured devil.....agape
Rejuvenated painful desire, enforces youthful
vigour
Perfect tears form
In crystallised abstracted absurdity
Loves dying passion, seduces my logic
In negative obscurity
Violently thousands die
In selfish love

Exerted
Ocean of death.

Loves' Suicidal Embrace

Brittle crimson frosted lips
Pout crumpled delirious desire
Whirlpool of emotions dance and divide
Oceanic fingers lacerate my heart
Mouthed pearls of headless love
Flesh of no-flesh dies, dies and dies
For the love of love of love, the love of you

Sacrificial smiles eye your cold glow
Peaches ignite our mirrored embrace
Disfigured pale blackness sparkles
Suffused tingling wantonness burns
Cusped breast teases my loins
Flesh of no-flesh dies, dies and dies
For the love of love of love, the love of you

Listening florets lash swirling chiffon
Deathless swimming corpuscles devoured
Bacterial growth, you on me in me-love

Disease of disease is my suicide-crucified
Nail me to your heart, heartless heart-love
Flesh of no-flesh dies, dies and dies
For the love of love of love, the love of you

Trample my corpse forlorn muse
Muddied but cleansed oysters naked
Scented and anointed with your love
Being in being, breath of breath, breathes
Rancid freshness enlivens my spirit of you
Flesh of no flesh dies, dies and dies
For the love of love of love, the love of you

Loves suicidal embrace is you-love
You, you and you, I die for you-my love, my love.

Melting Molasses.

The bee in your eyes
I sip sweetly
Your petal breasts
I envelope
Chestnut lightened hair
I dancingly caress
As sunlessly you burn!

Shadowless shadow
I follow darkly
Sheeted sky enembers me
Fingers fleshing your outline
Traced as tasted air-breathes
Meteors course the heavens
Glacial warmth melts me

Drunken with your dew
I slip into your lips
Reddened poppies-opiates of death

I am honey dripping.......
In cloudless trees.......
Wind kisses silently soundly
Meadows of summers-evaporate

As you part but am here
Me of me of you of me, is you
My hearts in yours-empty
Absence in non-absence
Is hollow of hollow in hollowness
Solidity is illusional nowness
Timeless time is seared in you, my bee.

Minds Enslavement-Skulled Boneless Love

Ego's construction company-defended, bloodied
river
Habituated thinking-experienced cyclic motion
Burdened I and I-encompass the sun of suns
Figurative lips stitched-speechless dried cactus,
deserted
Embedded fleshless heart-immolated in
lustfulness
Heedless intoxication-numbed emotional scars
Bag of diseased love-disillusioned youth of all
youths
Eyes poisonous possessiveness-suffocating in
beautiful ugliness
Equatorial amniotic fluid-fills earthen ears, the
sound of reason
Trembling fragile innocence-sacrificed genes,
forefathers sins
Knowledge burnt-raining corrosively, delusional
illusion

Razor embraced tree-skinned clouds, tinned logic

Ignorant indigestible life-tortured dusty wings, blown clean

Loves crumbling psyche-detached sensitivity, reality

Bursting blossoming compassion-flowered suffering

Pollinated fertile wisdom-seeded future, released

Prisoner of prisoners-no more

Liberation is all-universal law

Beginning of beginnings-end of all ends is;

LOVE FOR ALL.

Mirror of Awareness, Heart of Compassion

To be and not be, in autistic apelessness, apeingly
aping
The unawareness of unlanguage is the language
of love
My eyes, yours in the mirror of kindness, hearts
swim singingly
The burka of awareness, scented lips-unspoken
joyfulness's joyless joy
Purities hairless child, touching cheeks-kissed
roses, tender blissfulness
Dolls valley beacons, sedated nightless
nightmares stampeded heart
Suns breasts warming branches of enfolded you,
humblingly humble
Moon carouses, skies coarseness washes
shoeless stars of darkness's dark lotus's golden
mud, ecstatically dances in clarified clarities clarity
of unclarity

Boddhi tree's seedless seeds, compassionate
compassion flowers in your smile
Ants wander in pathless paths view of non-views
view in its viewless view of non-view

Moon's Fruitless Shadow

The sheets of your flesh, embrace;
The flower of my eyes breathless caress
Frailties shadow, memorises your blossoming
scent
Swimming lifeless clouds of seductive snowflakes;
Melt in my mouth's spineless kiss of no kiss, but to
kiss
Tasting the knowledge of your wombless head of
no head
Starfish ears listen to, bloodied grey faceless
expression
Wheat curves around your golden bosom, bread
of no bread
Swaying nipples drink of my lust, petals bathe my
awareness
Treading gentle sandy space, atomless hair
breathes-virtues
Rainbows film skates across, heartless moon's
savannah

Tears soak my breast, pollinating my mind with
painful doubt
Saffron's autumn rock traverse's consciousness's
loveless light
Cranes beckon waterfalls fernless moss-misty
heavens release
Sundews enfolding carnivorous embrace
devourers hearts

Nightshade Mirrors Freedom

The converged eyes mirror the nightshade of
rageless death
Harpy eagle rips chattering minds chains of
deceitful flowers
Brittle urchin bodilessly walks the Judas tree of
snakeweed
Lacewings entombed delicacy drunk, puffer fish's
spinney ego
Descended flycatcher sawlessly face's the
portraiture of pain
Mosquitoes probe chambers of quatrain's mafia
cellophane cage
Bacteria suffuses minds scattered effluence of
walled silence
Vines clambering throat delirious bacchanal
chasm cheated
Wrathful antenna taste decayed wheels of
spiralling dejection

Pithless sun freckles earths molten embryonic felt spa

Pampas laughingly dries ice, centuries splintered lagoons

Fleeting skylarks stream in declining rock faces shadow

Fathoms hallowed sacrificial calcite bubbles energetically

Elasticised poisons vie dominantly in crouched cities

Conspired cathedrals jostle in chivalrous debasement

Crucified ass kisses the oasis of heraldries cunning

Hedonism bathes in moonlights bloodied floor

Bridged palms of diamonds, dredge the sullied soul

Kibbutz of laboured fruit, planted toil of aggression

Dwarfed logic towers in disintegration of lectern

Burning visions of flesh elevated to oceanic delight

Perseverance preserved in withered chattering

Leafless awareness dies in sand dunes of Spartan
surf
Reign of lotus jewels the heavens in desireless
light
Clouded phial of changeling morphs the valleys
Vagabond of warlords decreased humidity-expired
Axis of weaponry consumes aconites eye-
bloomed
Nobility humbly drinks lecherously the leper's
wisdom
As the end of all ends is no-end, but beginingless
endlessness.

Oceans of Emptiness.

The breathless expanse of dharmadhatu
Jewels of obscience shine wishfully granting
Clarity of spaciousness
In fields of dhayani Buddha's

Ornaments-Trinkets of Love.

I wear the garland of death
Opening men's hearts and eyes, grief
Tears of tranquillity-mother Ganga
Bodily trinkets-hearts, loves, memories;
Others-soul captivators, ensnarers-Mara
Ornaments of sound-scattered, lost-forever
present
The "om" "ah" of sacred space, soundlessly
devoid
The flowering, "you," "me," "us"-of nothing
Selfless, energies-starless light
The cobra's fire, is my rain-love
Shelter of non shelter-fearlessly loving
Painless pain is the pain of attachment-other
I am the fisher of souls, captivator of captivated
minds
I have yours, my flower, listening hearts,
whisperings
The gesture of non-gesture, the breeze

The caress of caresslessness;

The breathlessly breathing, the wind

Oh bliss of blisslessness, blissful dance of endless
time

In and of the universe-our beginnings;

Our ends, touching joy, of the bliss Queen,

Tara,

Tara's, love.

Painful Loveless Curse-Freedom

Life's heart felt..........detritus
Cursed to live a loveless life!!

Mother O mother destroyer
Destroy me with your darkest love
Nefarious weapons sharpened
Cut off the head of hope
Abandonment, she pierces my heart
Severed hands, not able to grasp;
Tenderly touching soft flesh, lips
Wear the girdle of selfless non-attachment
String together mindless heads
Beautiful garland adorns your neck
Bloodied black breasts, swaying
Mount my limbless, headless corpse
Mother desire extinguish my passions
In blissfully surrendered body
Destroyer of delusional reality
Blackest of voids illuminates;

Enlightened Love and Wisdom,

Freedoms heart found!!!

Pain-Love Dichotomy

Body seared flesh, companionship
Mind-intellectual seductive tormenter
Emotional pain-learn to love your own tears
Taste the bitter sweet, as memories trickle
Joyous face faces amnesiac, hating world
Suicide-bomber walks in barren loveless realm

Ready to let go!

Depersonalised, dehumanised fragmented self
Explodes-implodes

Outcaste

Dalit
Nigger
Jew
Tibetan
Palestinian

Brother Sister, oppressed, depressed

Dispossessed

Gather-join hearts join hands

Selfless love, for other............the torturer,

Will heal your own pain
And the worlds!

Embrace your heart
And;
Love
Practice love
Endless love

However-painful.

Possession 2nd

"Nick" someone shouts from behind, he turns to look but all he sees are disjointed shadows amongst neon-clouded streets. Loneliness hits him like a sheet of ice as midnight creeps in, he wanders off down the main road until he comes to a sprawl of Hazelnut trees, he collects the empty husks and puts them into his bag, mixing with stones and Chinese coins. Suddenly a car flashes on its head lights. Has he been exposed? He'd better go; secrecy is all, as he rushes of into the black sticky tar with amber screeching above him. Something beckons him up a fire escape, four floors in all as he stands at the top. "Shall I jump?" he asks himself. He sways in the wind, his stomach turns as he shakes with the rush of adrenaline. "I can't," he mumbles to himself. Slowly he clambers down to scamper off home. The moon calls, the red door entices him in, up the stairs, blinded by negativity he staggers to bed, he can't sleep as thoughts wash around his head like billions of stars in the universe.

Dawn has come. Merlin pours him into the Holy Grail he scours paragraphs underlined, they speak a strange tongue, he becomes transfixed for hours as the words have a personal tinge, the air lies pregnant with darkening madness. He cooks some saffron rice, the plate lies on the floor, a harsh shout from inside tells him to piss on it. He devours it with animal lust; he showers the walls with this potion. Visions of the pentagram in the cellar flash into his mind, he stands on his feet, a force of immense strength tries to suck him through the wall, he turns and heads for the door, evil resides here, must get away. He falls down the stairs, out into the open.

He floats down the road, "must call someone, anyone," he thinks to himself. Two cars collide with a loud bang, twisted together like a pair of lovemaking octopuses, the other growls at him; he keeps walking, following his nose to who knows where. Shattered faces glare at him, he looks for signs scraped into brickwork and on the pavement, a car revs up but there is no driver, headlights burn and leave holes in his body. He comes to terms with a body that is not his, how many others live in here he asks himself, is he possessed is the question, where can he get help?

A church. Maybe a priest can help. There on the hill is a giant toad, eyes pointing up towards heaven. He ponders, "Is God an alien?" Which speck of dust did he come from? He gets nearer, gargoyles gape in disbelief, he walks through the doors of an open wound of oak and iron, blackened with years of sinners' stains of conscience. A font of holy water hangs off the wall like a mothers breast bursting with milk, it burns his forehead, the noise from the street makes him twitch as he enters the abyss, his footsteps echo to a song of silence. There above the alter, Jesus hangs on a cross ten feet wide, he passes under it, energy falls through him with the weight of centuries, he crumbles like stale bread into a heap on the floor. Broken splintered thoughts scurry in despair to find a place in his head. "Its not safe here." He thinks to himself. He melts down the path to his flat, it begins to rain, are these tears of love washing the world clean? He climbs into bed wet and dirty. Dreams buffet him from corner to corner until daylight eventually arrives. He looks at the clock; its late afternoon, coffee and a fag are all he needs. The kitchen has been redecorated in saffron rice, despair punches his teeth out as smoke fills the room, desperately he thinks to himself he must find a priest. Darkness closes the curtains on the day. He panics as he stumbles out the door and up the road to the Seven day Evangelical church. Poisoned with fear and dread he enters the citadel of stone and wood. A black man approaches, he sobs incoherently that he's possessed. Can they help? Yes comes the reply, twelve in all link hands together, but he is the thirteenth, Judas. They sing, he burns his leg starts to shake violently. Black energy moves down and enters the earth. Tears stop, is he cleansed? He feels delicate, they release him, he slowly enters the street. "Free at last!" he shouts, he looks at the ground, then a black cloak descends. He thinks it hasn't worked; death is the only answer, to end it all he must die.

Profoundly Beautiful-Madness.

Let me kiss your eyelids, your frosted lips, and
your crescent breast's!
Pools smilingly beam-opalescent dusty pearls-
moonlight
Lashes, freckled cheeks-bend the ignited
glistening stair's
She, bloodlessly intoxicates-scented flower of
tears-pressed
Bleakly howling winds-excitingly shakes my heart-
fractured
Creepers bracingly seep through limbless stance-
floating
She-wolf, stalks treeless fodder-reflected
night...............glow's
Lungless blizzard, scorched snow-flaked skin-
melts,
Fleshless memories, rattling bones, deceived
territory

Landless land, marches nowhere-drowning battlements

Maps of no maps, finds her;

Tattered wings, brittle doors, sealed waxen mind's-escape

Labyrinth of desires, Minotaur of thought, pursued reflection

Shattered faecal translucent joy, breastless sun-cools

Hidden womb, throned-King of Kings, relentless sea

Swallowed pride, humilities consumed…………dust-cloven bed

Ploughed field, seedless fertility-silken cloak, liquid light

Golden birth, oblivions shore, totemic dance……..wreathed love

Pollinated being, sprinkled bliss, foetal-rainbow's matrix

Birth of no birth's, primal scream's echo, corridor of trainless train

Movement of no movement, cycling
stillness…………….. knotted contemplation
Ringed Psilocybin, waif………eye`s vulnerable
giants-underbelly, softened greed
Worthless treasure,
nothingness……………priceless primeval mud-
stirred
Purities blossom, Lotus Lake, fireless water of fire,
bathed naked awareness………..
Blind vision, sees the seer, crystal gaze,
translated darkened light-eclipsed
Wholeness-grained clarities sand, hours of
seconds, slip through her hands
Totalities shadow follows, silhouetted walls, gated
fountain-sensed……..shelled sound
Wisdoms beauty dazzle`s-profound madness-
reality revealed……………….. and loved!

Rain of the Day

Despairingly eyes blur-friends, lovers, enemies
Droplets hanging from cloudiness's clouds
Pollutions evaporating-raining days shadows
Washing earth's stillness to source
Ebbing and flowing-moonless friend's cycle
Seashore of the unsure-unsurity of doubtless
doubt
Youthful fountains-sagging baggage of life, history

Regurgitated Matter

Black light-holed, crushed hollow spirit

Saturn devours his children, endless seconds-split

Green lion swallows sunshine's wholeness-fruited breasts

Timeless time of no time-ceaseless nothingness, beginingless end

Plant, absorbed light-chlorophyll batteries fuelled-seeded generation

Oxygen chewed-bloody nourished flesh-vanities survival

Carbon-beginingless diamonds-building blocks, universal desire

Limes deconstructed calcium-framed, scaffolding-exoskeleton's revenge

D.N.A.`s ladder-X & Y, Jacobs's history remembered-fleeced riches

Exploded, imploded, super nova-worlds spinning endlessly spiralling

Space dust, cosmic soup, stirred senseless trivia-
crowned poverty
Methane ignites Pandora's and Agni`s heart-
stolen chaos
Vampire sucked soulless matter-zombie's hatred-
fractal's blossoming
Intercourse of exchanged language-uprooted blind
knowledge
Edit, juggle-philosophical debate-eschewed
brains-forked tongue
Garbage of recycled psychiatrist-medicated
slumber-blinkered rational
Digest, kill-sustained beings-endless destruction-
consumerism
Kali-suffused light, purified winds-cornered globe
quartered
Sea of tranquillity-godless moon, wars of jealous
placental madness
Iron smoldering-axeless tissues, hammered ears
of wheat-staple sound

Sarcophagus-flowered joy-beautiful earthen
wealth, returning source
Blood stained soil-instinctual fertilised
consciousness-reaped foundations
Radiated death sustained-humans meaninglessly
swirl-skulled wasteless mass
Worm of idea, infinity gracelessly grasped-
bafflement, profoundly illuminates
Addled reality-senseless matter absorbed-life's
nonsensical mess, exchanged
Bastardised goddess of no god, spacious space-
expansionless atoms-dissolved
Accelerated collision of lives, synchronistically
energised...............all for what?
Regurgitated matter-fact......why of birth-life
is.........endlessly spawned-nonsense!

Rimpoches Musical Awareness.

My heart is the breath in your flute

My lungs are your hands

My eyes are your dreams;

In your dreamless stateless state of

dreamlessness

My limbs are your thoughts

My arms your love

My bones your karmic framed history

My flesh your sustenance

My hair your windless wisdom

My nails your broken heart

My feet your compassionate gait

My fingers your earth

My secret place yours in desire

My belly your temple in supplication

My kidneys your purifier

My nose your fragrance of skin

My ears the resounding silence of you

My memories the dusty butterfly of your space

My breast yours to tear and cry on

My buttocks yours to grow hardened

My headlessness is in yours, heedlessly

My mind floats through your desert

My pores your release in excess

I swim in you for you, I am you.

Shadowless Shadow

Shadowless shadow floats along paths
Mist seeps through moss covered branches
Ladened heart washes down the stream,
endlessly
Bloodied tears quench the soil of decomposition
Zested fruit maggot encrusted rind, rolls
unknowingly
Declining incline of angler fish, tempted and
teased
Baited darkened love, suffused nothingness`s
silhouette
Fleshless soft skin, phantom's embraced
disgraced smile
Moons waning, lustre of longing dies in a puddle
Masked ugliness surveys beauties blossom
dirtiness
Captured, she tears his wings into tissues of grief
Airlessly buoyant he scrapes the depths of desire

Nature's denuded papyrus, parchment of history sealed

Fleetingly escaping between bladeless lilies-sunless

Legless limbs fingered crevices, cobwebbed back

Algae's cotton breathes-deoxygenated cortex

Bubbleless thought intoxicatingly dives into cobalt

Handless door of no-door, hinges greased rusty gas

Acidic detritus, tanned clouds of batik-swallowed

Meandering eyes seduce sirens dulcet tones-languid

Straw covered breasts squared-enflamed wind rages

Cuckoo spit enfolds nettles grasp-smokey alter risen

Ribbon of swords swavering blizzards, bitingly snatched

Frosted meadows prison scented corpse calls closer

Leprosy's tower chimes in cavernous gorge-
whispered
Gossamer cloaked days, entombed slimeless
nightingale
Elderberries fertility wines in couched silence
Bracken entwined, kisses encapsulated barrow
Cairn scattered meridian of boundaries-measured
Shadowless night of shadows, steals icily away
As no human casts darkness in essence!

Silken Swords

Attachment to what is past is as;

The crazy fool gluing a broken pot
With the bespoken tongue, deplete
Of spittle, the healing wind,
The breathe of love, life's hearts;
The silken shadow, knives of a thousand eyes;
Can not pierce karmic protection;
Flesh on bones;
Retribution,
The reign of the five poisons, subjugate to;
Gardens of light, forever present………………
Silken swords cut through Maras blinding arrows
Assailing the love beyond all love, compassion;

For all, is this not attachment, the thorn of love

Thunderous vibrancy, oceans of realities in a
pearl,

Universal flowers, the light of love…..beginnings in
non-beginnings;

Attached to attachments, who labels who?

In the vehicle of expression,
Language the breathe of action;
An act of violence, to breathe
Is there a need………………an attachment, the
kiss

To the light of sightlessness, retribution/revenge,
For one smitten to dust, is a fool's heart so foolish;
In irresponsible attachments, the lies of fabricated
suffering,
Blinding others, the "rolang" of Sin Poi's medicine,
The blue beryl of directed attachments, is this
wisdom?
Attachments, unchanging karma, ripe and unripe,
compassion;

Attachments to silk, the silken sword of
compassion
Cuts with the breath, caresses of gentle eyes,
love,
Love.

Stones of Labyrinthine Warmth

I draw the lawn with my feet, as attention worms into the suns braided clouds, sandy blood fuels the fleshless tree of doubt, moons eclipsed heart swims in a field of daisy breasted earth, swaying chains of glass support pillars of duplicated starfish listening to darkness's feathers heavier than love, floating down egoless voided avenues of quantum ethereal vessels, absorbing lungs of concrete, tarmac skin faces irradiated showers of dreamless rainbows as muddied captains plot a ring of mushroomed halo's, limbs of planets jostle universe's scented treasure, dustless breath of oceanic delightful daffodils, blasted thoughts drink visions past of presentless genetics, milked sanity kisses the depth of no depth, hills fingered eyes glisten on the horizon of skulled spores, drifting arms embrace the emptiness of emptiness, the form of formless form, seeping tears submerged in reef of barren nourishment skipping on galaxies of hairless pregnancy added and subtracted divided and divided fraction of algebraic minuet calls from sunsets curved umbilical of supplied frosted nitrogen of turquoise flowers trodden and sodden with allies of grandiose shoes of no shoes, twenty seventh heaven dying to burn the undergrowth with agents of brackish water in motion, sloughing wounds sapping insects of convexed being, tumbling laughter follows the fallow trough of ploughed pain seeded with mustards atom, deathless smiles paced mechanisms objectifies the object of objection of no objection to subjection, paralleled perception sinks in clarities lotus warmth as voice of no voice pierces the temple of sacrificial longitude of dualistic courtship in dances of energetically teased fondness of helium filled skies of cusped conversation bartered and fed for no price-except love, washed ego anoints the she, the she of love, the she of wisdom, the she of beauty, the she of filth, the she of ugliness, the she of creativity, the she of cruelty,

the she of famine, the she of the universe-love,
the love of no love, yet love, love.

Su Ti`s Petals

Tears, icicles dancing desirously

Chasms of darkened joy-lovelessly loving

Destroyer of heart lines meet-kissing nightshade

Sun's softened ecliptic woman, milked-painlessly

Sacrificial pen, quilted mysticism-poetess's theatre

Saffron, persimmon smoked-suttee's calligraphy
honoured

Children of phamaldahides whiskey-boundlessly
bonded

Treeless words echo in buddlia's dragon vetch
valley

Monkfish's fatness, cancerous suicidal silence,
silenced

Breached reservoirs of karmic skies-fallen clouds
walk endlessly

Skinless monitor scurries in communicating desert
oasis of dryness

Divided nomads of choiceless choice-libated gods
whisper

Daughters empty head, heading eastward in kabuki of No
Folded tea of infused Geisha's heartless heart-worshipped
Trains of silken moths, golden textured water-weaved love
Lakshmi`s temples of wavering light-ignited butter, moulded
Conifers reddened seedless Pict`s-scolded prosperity deflowered
Jaguar's stealthy Newtonian eye, dusting dust's flavourless flavour
Odious odes of Oedipal grapes, stampeding warrior's buried-china
Wombed stars of gypsies filtering purities roses-scattered petals
Enriched heartened soil, poetess's wisdom-denuded joy, joyfully joyless.

Subjugated Heart of Heart

Assassinated lovers memories

Ragged fingernail wrenched grief

Corpse of enslavement, bound

In intestinal coiled wrists

Bloodied shameless face

Blackened suns dismembered lies

Bodied cleaved chest, plucked

Flowering aorta swallowed

Dirtied sullied soiled breath

Consumed foetal love

Dies in bondage of maternal hatred

Sweet Corrosive Innocence

Eyes feathered limb scorches my skin
Corrosive fingers, explore my mouth
Tongue meets tongue in saliva's explosive
massage
Raw venison, kisses my encapsulated breast
Honeyed cusped nipples, arrested in supplication
to the sun
Bonded heart suffocates in lustful boiling sweat
Drowning delirious depravity, I fall at the alter
Bloodied teeth mesmerisingly encase his member
Shameful gaze, ecstatic head, gyrating supernova
Imploding black hole, vacuum sealed bodies
Flayed child's innocent breath
Released in anthraxes decomposed embrace
Bleached bones, solicit scattered remains
Death's hunger absolved, once again.

The Absence!

Totalities absent heart, degraded
Rendered walls, loosest of touch
Drowned gardens flowerings
Being of non-being jumps
Purple maggot, devouring its innards in denial
Twisted corrosive love-breathes haplessly
Sullied sodden petrifaction-wrapped `n clothed
Fearful hunger cries aloud in silences cage
Wanton nothingness abandons hope
Something of nothing is something!
Crimson breast-bleeds in famines richness
Throat catch of green world-denuded
Pirated radio sweetens the crowded air
Waves sway in absence of crested Grebe
Indian summer infuses the horizon-smokelessly
Windows of longing tick onwards, at silhouettes
Guarded journeys cattled memories, blown to dust
Spring boxes with snapdragons cycle of bitterness
Gorges of gorgon in ravines of solitaire,

Flowingly she meanders in amusement

Earthen shrimp scurries to boiling point

Stairingly the stars hurtle towards the night sky

Rabbit of dis-eased birth, culled inlet reddened

Painful simplicity of blackness-eyes the universe

Snatched tree twinkles in deathless embrace

Primed and coated suicide, bombs outward

Corridors of blighted light-blinds the day

Koala, skinned tobacco chewed and spat at

Measured absence inches in metric rhythm

Beaten heart felt egg, cracked corn sniffed

Steamed essence vegetates at peppered moon

Blissfully tender grass-foddered thinking cut

Miraculously the absence of desire is desired

Lepers salmon chimes and gurgles at thought

Centrality of perfume ignites my vision

Lingerie drifts in endless sea of freshless flesh

Beaches of hairless palms coded tropics captured

Glistening scythe of mirrored puddle-beckons

Quickening sands quiver in the lightness of;

The Absent absence is no absence is absent;

The absence of endless nothingness is;
Absent.

The Cathedral of Chaos.

Spectre of chaotic light dissolves
In a cathedral of coralline beauty
Atoms collide in damaged exchange
Absorption of scared tissues, scavenged
Fleshes ravaged bones, boiled down
Supplication to the bards of death
Stained glass shrouds the sunlight
Temple of blackened day scorched
Market sellers lament bloodied vision
Hourless figurine gargoyles the reign
Arched spineless gallows of hatred
Flex the muscles of stone cornered
Amassed bemusement of singular space
Edging toward the framework of darkness
Eclipsed death of radical design snuffed
Fleeced mentality, coat of other shielded
Emblematic roses of white and red
Joust and jostle in turmoil of estuarine waters
To breathe the sporeless fertility of decomposition

Weakened life, changeling of confused di-spire`s

Infinities chains hammered out, painful forgery

Snapshot of non-existence imprisoned dome

Jailers of paradise entombed love unrewarded

Ransomed being of sterling's quickness shot

Poisonous flowers blossom in consumerism

Altercation of sacrificial desire challenged

Vanities benchmark examined and executed

Headless seduction of swamped hearts

Denuded jealousy, transposed eyes vie;

In labyrinthine of centralities wombed breast

Deathlessly dancing in histories clothes

Searing vision of purity, exposed vulnerability

Initiation in her kiss, the kiss of rebirth

And dies in the cathedral of chaos.

The Cloudlessness of Joyfulness

The cloudiness in your eyes, sodden with the grief of love, hearts floating between dusk and dawn, light softens my flesh as your breath tingles my spine, arms move as cotton swaying in the southern fields, budding in the depths of your warm breasts, sun nourishes your divine curvaceousness, flowing misty hair of Leander's entwining leafless lashes fluttering in absence of dewless flower surrounding rootlessness of surf splashing our skins, wading into the blue of non-blue, she smiles softening my ardour inflaming my loins and heart, we tumble airlessly leaching expansiveness's stars, melting in a buttery embrace spreading out in grey concrete pavements, delicate feet humbly imprinting, in a circumambulation of islands in a swave of palm trees riding the blackened despair of ignorance's sandlessness, until our dust is frozen in the timelessness of time, constructed particles heedlessly rushing arriving no-where but somewhere, chasing rainbows of rainbows but of no-rainbows as your colourful fullness, endlessness of endless goalessness descending in an ascendance of blissful joy, limb reaching limblessly in love, your coat, your bath, your fire-lips that cannot speak, but speak of your Shadowless shadow following a trough of betrovements opening the window to your sky, to glance at you is to pierce the chill of night washing the moons barren fertility ebbing at your shore returning with the magnetism of your love, but to die in the dropless ocean of oceanlessness`s ocean, is to love in a dreamless dreamlessness of dreamless dreaming of no-dream but dreamingly dreaming of dreamlessness, is to live in love.

The Converged Eyes Mirror the Nightshade of Rageless Death

The converged eyes mirror the nightshade of
rageless death
Harpy eagle rips chattering minds chains of
deceitful flowers
Brittle urchin bodilessly walks the Judas tree of
snakeweed
Lacewings entombed delicacy drunk, puffer fish's
spinney ego
Descended flycatcher sawlessly faces the
portraiture of pain
Mosquitoes probe chambers of quatrain's mafia
cellophane cage
Bacteria suffuses minds scattered effluence of
walled silence
Vines clambered throat delirious bacchanal chasm
cheated
Wrathful antenna taste decayed wheels of
spiralling dejection

Pithless sun freckles earths molten embryonic felt
spa

Pampas laughingly dries ice, centuries splintered
lagoons

Fleeting skylarks stream in declining rock faces
shadow

Fathoms hallowed sacrificial calcite bubbles
energetically

Elasticised poisons vie dominantly in crouched
cities

Conspired cathedrals jostle in chivalrous
debasement

Crucified ass kisses the oasis of heraldries
cunning

Hedonism bathes in moonlights bloodied floor

Bridged palms of diamonds, dredge the sullied
soul

Kibbutz of laboured fruit, planted toil of aggression

Dwarfed logic towers in disintegration of lectern

Burning visions of flesh elevated to oceanic delight

Perseverance preserved in withered chattering

Leafless awareness dies in sand dunes of Spartan
surf
Reign of lotus jewels the heavens in desireless
light
Clouded phial of changeling morphs the valleys

The Death of a Thousand Deaths is no Death, but Death

To embrace death is to love life, the life of death

To die in the mirror of stupidity, is to face deaths'
face

Burning cold hell is supreme death, the death of
wisdom

Wisdom dies as she is born; the death of no death
is death

Decayed reality, death in the moment is no death
of death of death

Death renews her conceit at herself-death, death
eyes death squarely

Death dances as she is deathlessly deathless in
the death-no death

To love is to die; deathless beauty is the death of
deathlessness of no death

She whores her progeny, the birth of no birth is
deaths birth of death

Deaths currency is the prosperity of poverty, the wealth of poverty, death

Death wears the finest jewels and ornaments-superficiality of wealthlessness

She brazenly walks nakedly clothed, honoured and renovated-enshrined

She is the resurrection of birthless death of birth, she is your guarantee

Holding her hand in marriage is the love of each moment in the death of death

To love death is to awaken in life; the death of life is the life of life-deathless death

She is constantly reborn, but unborn in birth of no birth of death is birth-death

She is you and not you but me and not me, to live is to love her but not love her

We reject her but can not forget her, oh how we wish!

Blow out her candle and die, as death is to live in her-the womb of death is life,

Death.

The Grief of Life, Wellspring of Eternity

She pours her heart out to replenish the earth!

Echoless beings, once were-resound in silence
Energy of no-energy worms into the black void
The pain of birth of rebirth of no-birth of birth
What is love but stone parchment-inklessly written
Connection of no-connection of connections
absorbed
Intertwining roots and branches suffused in
deathlessness
Barren fertility of desert roses-petrified sun of
basilisk's stares
Tanneries drunkenlessly stained tea ceremony-
honoured
Rice paper flesh of no-flesh, tortured tissue of
sixes & eights
Boundary of no-boundary is the edge of
edgelessness-nothingness

Pulse of magnetic screeching-attracted
compassionate heir-encircled
Embryonic embroidered particles-scatter the
shatterless spaciousness of no-space
Neptune stirs the universe with the Styx of
nameless pain, of no-pain but gain
Cloaked invisibility of chiffoned breast-heartless
life of loveless love-life
Lichens leached-in threshold of golden fragment
of encapsulated minor
Famines banquet emboweled in cannibalistic rite
of a danceless rhythm
Dried wellspring of pruned whispers lashes the
shore of turtles' nests
To begin, the grief of no-grief is the loveless grief
of love-eternity.

The Moon

You bore through your hips
Milky white moon
Oh, daughter to the stars
Dusty time has disfigured you
Left you barren and bare

Fated to hug the earth
My blood ebbs and flows
As you appear and disappear
I die a milky white death

You're a guide in the dark
When love's light is low
Because you torment me so
Dying each month and being born anew

The Net of Deceit

I am not

A knot of the netting of;

Otherliness`s other, the mirror

Ensnared desire, netted deceit

Figurine moves in blind alleys

The net of the periphery;

Of you, me, non ness of one ness

Shivite of lyres, universal vibrations

The beat of atoms, atomically numbered

Numerologies of deceitfulness, emptiness

The heart is voided of and in lightness

The flower wilts, the perfume entraps

The browed plough of parallelograms

Your furrowed breasts, beacons of memories

The pinnacle of enriched attachments

The net caste, fathomless dalits scarcity

My bidding is your bidding,

Oh mirror of deceit, illusionary magician

I attach to non ness the spaciousness of;

Deceits net, Mara the ensnarer.

The Sugar Cube

Forensics of faith
Crucify the crucifixion of;
Taste of taste........ yourselves
Tainted uniformnalities of;
Butchery......exposure of pigeon's dung
The Deng of penal servitude
Livers chow mien, gloating evil
Oesophagus of conveyor belt diplomacy
Sharpened feet, the axis of evil
Pencilled eyes, once valid;
No longer a commodity for truth
Commanded the risen corpses
Muffled tongues and stiletto siphoned life
Bones of you do, dancing for the sins of banshees
Negative sugar, the litmus for deathless life
Believe in lies the existence without existence
The butchery of social cohesion, guttered
Universal grief who's therapeutic God;
Do you call................ At the deal of the day

Child of mine the prison of non-ness

Suck baby suck the cored apple is reflected;

The ashen blacksmiths anvil bleeds

The legacy of the king's new cloths

Houses demolished for the piped mantle

Spare us some change guv……..

Saccharine youths dishevelled dried life

The black book the encounters of two

Alexandra bleats bloodied ears…………….

Silence speaks of truth without your lies,

Lesson in love…..I ask you Sugar cube

Faith in blindness…………my sweet.

The Thinness of Life's Soup

The thinness of life's soup is;
Realities kiss of unrealities normalness
Cosmically stirred muddiness
Impeaches the starlessness of stars
Imprinted barrenness, cannibalistic consumption
Desirelessly desiring egotistical worthlessness
Puddles of petroleum, tarred stupidity of extinction
Particle accelerates pressurised voided
punctuation
Politeness`s vulgarity of shallowness`s handshake
Is thinness to thin in its thickness of thinness?
Shaken compassion is the soupless gulags diet.
Chained whispers sing heartless beauty of
silence's
None other than tortured denial of denial to pray
Sacred grass spooned in its fatness of
vulnerability
Grandiose posturing of the posture of positionings
position

To point the view of veiwlessness of motions
motionlessness

Nobility of non-nobility in life's degradation of
acceptance

Anorexicness of thoughtless governmental
banners paraded

Watchlessly watching blankness of
uninterestingness`s interest

Eaten earthenness worms in sheepish bravery of
the herd

Singular multiplicity of non-singular singularity in
oneness

Bleached geography of chemical breathlessness
of breath

Sterile love of the famine of love in charitable
medallions

Instinctual drives the plough of destructions
fertilisation

Cloud burst doesn't wash bloodless life clean of
history

Racing racelessly to prejudicial correctness of incorrectness

Disciplines in ethical unmoralistic stems cellular cells imprisonment

The birth of rubbished birth discarded as soupless soups menu

The sale of limblesssness of life's guarantee of an unlife is guaranteed

Walled unity of curfewed intolerance as tolerance of unacceptance

To dine at the restaurant of life is the cheapness of wealthlessness`s worth

To love is to feast with beggars and whores the jewels of the heart

As dogs bark at the howling wind in its thinness of loveless life

To love is to swim in oceans of oceanlessness of to-days soupless soup.

The Voodoo Doll

A knock at the door
Open up
Laughter galore
A postman's gift
My sight has left me
Struggle to see
Bottoms and boobs
Its covered in nudes
I go inside
My Planet of the Apes
Has arrived
Frantically tear and rip
Nudes are not my trip
Curiosity has got
The better of me
I try to piece together
The torn parts
Suddenly it's a mass
Of blonde hair

I find a wax head

Then a leg

Torso to follow

But who is this broken doll

O voodoo doll

Is it me?

Heart and head

Who can tell?

Am I numbered?

As I awake

From my slumber

Ponder on and on

What does it mean?

The Vulgarity of Vagueness.

Crumbs of fragmented heart-tokens of doubt
Swept memories-scattered fleshlessness of;
Twigged-leafless bones-barren scientific
penetration
Desert's breast-milks lifeless love-dried parchment
Oasis of abandonment-red palms, drenchingly
sway
Dates for Christ-lack lustre jewels, sullied mud
Yoni of yogini-laughs at deathless void's embrace
Bowels of the abyss-altercated none starts blazing
Informationless information-blank book,
deforested;
Words-valueless meanings, deconstructed
interpretation
Library of vagueness-light of vulgarity, caviar
caned
Champagne of complexity-empty headed
universe, simplicity

Corked nipples-fathomless ocean-drowning brood
of jellyfish
Venomous loveless obscenity-coiled air heavy
with scentless must
Dreaded frozen polarity-fearless fear of
mathematical zero
Son of no sons is the sun, of deathless life-
radiated winds sear
Orpheus blindingly stumbles-Styx crossed-gallows
of forgetfulness
Goddess of criminality-stolen shrouded tender
hatred-remembered
Forged locksmith picked-intellectual juggled-naked
seasons evaporate
Brazen hearth-seaweed scattered bronze third-
eyed curvaceous rock
Pounded dolly-spindle of waves-friendship,
scuttled flight-gannet robed
Mouthed deafness, expressionlessly echoed
valley-cleaved Valhalla

Basilisk-petrified language-brailed golden oak-
vaulted heavens sealed
Metaphor erased-ashen Agni-blackened dayless
corpse-wormless composition
Saffron flayed cotton-fields sexlessly, cupped
cusp-divine water-burnt candy clay
Ambrosial feet kissed-decomposed bacterial
breath-freshened gilded moon-girdled warmth,
Equatorial furnished hips-carriage clock
accelerates-counting vagueness`s alarm!
Birth of wisdom-death of ignorant vulgarity-
vagueness dissolved-desire ended.

The Windswept Universe

The weeping skies tears of universal grief;
Waterfall of matter-human detritus recycled
Washed fleshless shores-the ebb & flow of love
Sunburnt eyes grieve for darkness's light
Atlas of universal grief-leaden heartless love
Embryonic womb of no womb-griefless grief
Grieving birth of no-birth is birth of birth of no-birth
Grief's breath caresses the skinless me of no-me
grief
To touch the joy of nature-is to grieve the grief of
grief
Beauty grieves for life, but grieves a deathless
grief
Grief's diamond sickle, the giver of life-grieves
To live is to grieve and to grieve is to live,
lovelessly
The grief of grief is no grief but the love to grieve
The freedom to live is the freedom to grieve-living
love

To grieve is to love-love deathlessly loving grief-
love
Windswept universe grieves of love in love to
grieve
Universal law is the law of no-law, to grieve!
The continuous continuum of no-continuum-grief
of love.

Tribute to Love and Pain.   (Dedicated to Louise)

I took the skies out of my heart
And saw the emptiness of the land

A drop of fire in the sea of love
Is the pain of life's barrenness?

Shrouds that walk the citadels of men's minds
Crying from the minuet of God's breath

Wombless child-a woman's eyes, condemned
To the stick of blindness's beggarliness`s hunger

A fountain's youth is the uterine garden of the
universe
Allah's man of twigs, the snap of sex-dustless dust

She of the red rivers of blackened earth's skyless
skies;

Are clouds, of icy doubt, the doubt of non-doubting
doubt?
Oh, to doubt-is to look into a woman's eyes, the
wind

The cheeks of the moons crumbling wings brush;
The picture of a painted you of non you-fleshless
flesh

Your why of why is the why of us,
Life's forest of words the fools ashen axe of
writing-corn

The plough share of your legs is the;
Supine sky of your lips-the kiss of the universe

The emptiness of your eyes, our breath
Is the cloak of your womb?
The cusped flowers of entwined grasses, last
season seasoning

The print of your life's shoes, is devoured in
history's timeless time
Our hearts the space of non space-love

The famine of your plastic breasts is;
Drunkenness's drunk
The nipple of listening waters-silence

Our matted belly, tied in equatorial mathematical
zeros of;
Zeus's pyre-the night of days daylessness is
today's day

The love of love of non-love;
Is the separation of non separation-us
To walk the voided void, is to meet in essence
To touch, to kiss, through spacious space of non
ness;
Is time's passage of non passage-us.
The weightless luggage of abandonment's
abandonment-love

Eons of eons can not extinguish;
The particle of us-love

Buttery flameless life
The lightened darkness's dark-us
Lightless light-love

The non-flame's flame is emptiness's emptiness
Your formless form in emptiness's form
Is the libation of self-arising liberation-love?

30/11/2004

Vaulted Heaven-She The Sky

Sky`s whirlwind eyes-blue of blue, but not blue
Dappled clouds-painted view-rides the Kingdom
Cotton lips kiss the sun-with each breathless
breeze
Skinned earth-shrouded love-watches gyratingly-
weights
Vaulted heart, charioteer of mind-milky arrows
pierced
Droplet of droplet-squeezed-freshlessly fresh;
Anointed body-libations smilingly-released
Embraced rainbow-bridges the metaphysical
Misty moss bites at shadows of lightless love
Trees nipple the horizon-lush hillocks roll
Ravines swimmingly hear-the moon's beckoning
Firing nightingales-whistling sand-dusty angels
Charcoal limbs-curvaceous streams-caress's
thighed estuary
Finger's spreading beach, cusp of ocean-girdles
hourglass compassion

Footprints left-timed dissolved, but not forgotten!
She of the Blue-Sky vaulted Heaven-ceaseless.

Wall of Words

Walls hide multitudes

Can't see, a rainbow, a mushroom

But not what you feel, faint quiver

Transparent eyes, burn through

Red brick heart

Naked black and white fleshed leaves

Brambleberry fingers glide along

Tess and Charlotte's spine

Silence squeezes down avenues of words

All in one momentary microcosm

Sectioned cruelty, magnified

Name by name, ordered thought

Desires roam free; screen, billboard

Subjective, ecstatic sensuality

Daily bread, infested language

Pollutants censor purity

Awkward aggression filters into streets of hate

Evil soup is on the modern menu

Love is terminated, onto the garbage heap of man

Can conscience release the spectre of the dead?

Politicians drown in moral decline

With a wall of words

Senseless.

Weavers of the sky.

She, vajrayogini-skydancer
Weaver of wisdoms essences
Blood drinker of compassion

Wild Yogini`s Endlessness of Endlessly Dancing, Dances.

Golden-breasted Dakini, moons smiling touchingly
felt
Anklets of voided wisdom resound in universal joy,
Dance of essences dancelessly dancing in
spacious spacious space
Gently support my chin with your vibrant warmth,
melting my lips
Belly bellows in wrathful graciousness with
starlight eyes, night sky
Swirling petals of reddened vajra umbrella,
beckons my ardour
Swaying fields of hair, oceanic corn of roughened
wildness of wildernesses
Laughter cuts directionless directions of "ha" in
slices of cloudless reality
Purity of skin the white of all whites is
beyondnesslessness of lotus feet

All eyes of concealed nothingness, nondualities
protectoress, echoes
Valleys ploughed in karmic painless pleasure,
fertility abounds barrenly
Hermitage of solitude is the boundarilessness of
nondifferentiality
The centre of centrelessness spiralling in infinities
love, the love of love
Oh mandalas of mandalas is spaciously aware of
unawareness of awareness
Embracing the embraceless embrace of grasping
at grasplessness is wisdoms heart.
Wild yogini dance the endless dance of
blissfulness`s joyfulness's spacious space.
1/09/2004

Worlds Within Worlds of Worldlessness`s Worldliness

Worlds colliding essences mixing converging
Worlds of sentient beings submerged in samsara
Deities of matter spirit within spirit-lifelessly alive
Atoms meeting across universalness, why of
where
What attracts also repels, collisions of condition
karma
Chemically charged interdependent threaded
existence
Negative and positive are worlds of non worlds-
denied
Dualistic non sense is sensed in senselessness of
senses
Worlds of gated gateless entrances of enterless
entrances
Flowers dancing in exchanged smiles of warmth of
gestures

Oceans of dropless universes of nothingness of
suchnesslessness
Sky goers walking in airlessness`s fire of water-
expansiveness`s space
Rock of non-rock is transpired in its transparency
of matterless matter
Misty breathless breath breathes the lightless light
of compassion
Goldenness is goldless golds gold melding to
formless form of Buddhahood
Letterless letters windlessness of blessings are
written but not written-penless
Invisibility of visibility is blinded sight of
sightlessness-searing sun's sunlessness
Manifesting in diseaseless disease's transformed
in blessed supplication of disirelessness
Humilities stallion glides across steppes in
stepplessness`s warrior of nobility of beggarliness
Bladeless bladed grass, Heruka of homeopathy
pierces the blackened heart of light

Rainbows manifest in dewless sky of skylessness
in crystalline clarities clarity
Timelessness is liberated in times timelessness of
time-mirrored in non-mirrorness
Charioteers plainnesslessness is redman's
nectarlessness of nectarless`s filthly purity
Worlds of non worlds of wordliness`s world is
fruitless fruit in guru's treeless tree
The spaciousness of spaceless space is
expasionlessnessly expanded expansion in
Emptiness of emptiness's emptiness in emptiness
is the risen formless form of form.

Wreaked on Love

Battered and bruised

Smashed against rocks

Craggy cove caresses my hull

As the waves of my tears

Splash and crash around my head

Thunderous roar

Masts splinter

Limbs broken

Lightening cracks

Sails shredded to strips

As my heart lies bleeding on the shore

Rocks bite and snarl

Like dogs at my keel

Barnacles crushed

Kelp wraps around my arm

I gulp for air

As love takes me under

Fish nibble

Drowning in love

Death of ego has come

What a wondrous feeling

Wreaked on love

www.ingramcontent.com/pod-product-compliance
Lightning Source LLC
Chambersburg PA
CBHW021158010426
R18062100001B/R180621PG41931CBX00024B/43